Everything You Need to Know About Diarrhea

Causes ♦ Symptoms ♦ Treatment

Watch a video version:
https://www.youtube.com/watch?v=R-8i4O5f6s8

This book is based on information and recommendations by the Department of Health, United States government.

Created By The Bizmove Health Team

AF439755

Disclaimer

All the content found in this book was created for informational purposes only. The Content is not intended to be a substitute for professional medical advice, diagnosis, or treatment. Always seek the advice of your physician or other qualified health provider with any questions you may have regarding a medical condition. Never disregard professional medical advice or delay in seeking it because of something you have read in this book.

ISBN: 9798748119054

Everything You Need to Know About Diarrhea

Diarrhea is loose, watery stools three or more times a day. Diarrhea may be acute, persistent, or chronic:

- **Acute diarrhea** is a common problem that typically lasts 1 or 2 days and goes away on its own.
- **Persistent diarrhea** lasts longer than 2 weeks and less than 4 weeks.
- **Chronic diarrhea** lasts at least 4 weeks. Chronic diarrhea symptoms may be continual or may come and go.

How common is diarrhea?

Diarrhea is a common problem. Acute diarrhea is more common than persistent or chronic diarrhea. Researchers estimate that about 179 million cases of acute diarrhea occur in the United States each year.

What are the complications of diarrhea?

Dehydration

Diarrhea may cause dehydration, which means your body lacks enough fluid and electrolytes to work properly. Your body loses more fluid and electrolytes in loose stools than solid stools. See a list of the symptoms of dehydration.

Malabsorption

Diarrhea may cause malabsorption. If people do not absorb enough nutrients from the food they eat, they may become malnourished. Certain conditions that cause chronic diarrhea—such as infections, food allergies and intolerances, and certain digestive tract problems—may also cause malabsorption. See a list of the symptoms of malabsorption.

What are the symptoms of diarrhea?

The main symptom of diarrhea is passing loose, watery stools three or more times a day.

People with diarrhea may also have one or more of the following symptoms:

- an urgent need to use the bathroom
- cramping
- loss of control of bowel movements
- nausea
- pain in the abdomen

People with diarrhea caused by some infections may also have one or more of the following symptoms:

- bloody stools
- fever and chills
- light-headedness and dizziness
- vomiting

Diarrhea may cause dehydration and malabsorption.

What are the symptoms of dehydration and malabsorption?

Dehydration and malabsorption can be serious complications of diarrhea. Their symptoms in adults, infants, toddlers, and young children are as follows.

Dehydration

Symptoms of dehydration in adults may include:

- thirst
- urinating less than usual
- feeling tired
- dark-colored urine
- dry mouth
- decreased skin turgor, meaning that when your skin is pinched and released, the skin does not flatten back to normal right away
- sunken eyes or cheeks
- light-headedness or fainting

Signs of dehydration in infants, toddlers, and young

children may include

- thirst
- urinating less than usual, or no wet diapers for 3 hours or more
- lack of energy
- dry mouth
- no tears when crying
- decreased skin turgor
- sunken eyes, cheeks, or soft spot in the skull

Malabsorption

Symptoms of malabsorption in adults may include

- bloating
- changes in appetite
- gas
- loose, greasy, foul-smelling bowel movements
- weight loss

Symptoms of malabsorption in infants, toddlers, and young children may include

- bloating
- changes in appetite
- gas
- loose, greasy, foul-smelling bowel movements
- weight loss or poor weight gain

Seek care right away

Diarrhea can become dangerous if it leads to severe dehydration. Diarrhea may also signal a more serious problem.

Adults

Adults with any of the following symptoms should see a doctor right away:

- diarrhea lasting more than 2 days
- fever of 102 degrees or higher
- frequent vomiting
- six or more loose stools in 24 hours
- severe pain in the abdomen or rectum
- stools that are black and tarry or contain blood or pus
- symptoms of dehydration

Older adults and adults with weakened immune systems or other health conditions who have diarrhea should also see a doctor right away.

Infants, Toddlers, and Young Children

The parent or caretaker of an infant, toddler, or young child with diarrhea and any of the following symptoms should seek a doctor's care right away:

- diarrhea lasting more than 24 hours
- fever of 102 degrees or higher
- severe pain in the abdomen or rectum

- stools containing blood or pus
- stools that are black and tarry
- symptoms of dehydration

What causes diarrhea?

Acute and persistent diarrhea may have causes that are different from those of chronic diarrhea. In many cases, doctors do not find the cause of diarrhea. Most diarrhea goes away on its own within 4 days, and finding the cause is not necessary.

Acute and persistent diarrhea

The most common causes of acute and persistent diarrhea are infections, travelers' diarrhea, and side effects of medicines.

Infections

Three types of infections that cause diarrhea include

- **Viral infections.** Many viruses cause diarrhea, including norovirus and rotavirus . Viral gastroenteritis is a common cause of acute diarrhea.
- **Bacterial infections.** Several types of bacteria can enter your body through contaminated food or water and cause diarrhea. Common bacteria that cause diarrhea include *Campylobacter* , *Escherichia coli* (*E. coli*), *Salmonella* , and *Shigella* .

- **Parasitic infections.** Parasites can enter your body through food or water and settle in your digestive tract. Parasites that cause diarrhea include *Cryptosporidium enteritis* , *Entamoeba histolytica* , and *Giardia lamblia* .

Infections in the digestive tract that spread through foods or drinks are called foodborne illnesses.

Infections lasting more than 2 weeks and less than 4 weeks can cause persistent diarrhea.

Travelers' diarrhea

Travelers' diarrhea is caused by eating food or drinking water contaminated with bacteria, viruses, or parasites. Travelers' diarrhea is most often acute. However, some parasites cause diarrhea that lasts longer. Travelers' diarrhea can be a problem for people traveling to developing countries.

Side effects of medicines

Many medicines may cause diarrhea. Medicines that may cause diarrhea include antibiotics , antacids containing magnesium, and medicines used to treat cancer.

Chronic diarrhea

Some infections, food allergies and intolerances,

digestive tract problems, abdominal surgery, and long-term use of medicines can cause chronic diarrhea.

Infections

Some infections from bacteria and parasites that cause diarrhea do not go away quickly without treatment. Also, after an infection, people may have problems digesting carbohydrates such as lactose or proteins in foods such as cow's milk, milk products, or soy . Problems digesting carbohydrates or proteins can prolong diarrhea.

Food allergies and intolerances

Allergies to foods such as cow's milk, soy, cereal grains, eggs, and seafood may cause chronic diarrhea.

Lactose intolerance is a common condition that may cause diarrhea after eating foods or drinking liquids that contain milk or milk products.

Fructose intolerance is a condition that may cause diarrhea after eating foods or drinking liquids that contain fructose, a sugar found in fruits, fruit juices, and honey. Fructose is added to many foods and soft drinks as a sweetener called high-fructose corn syrup.

Sugar alcohols such as sorbitol, mannitol, and xylitol may cause diarrhea in some people. Sugar-free candies and gum often include these sugar alcohols.

Digestive tract problems

Digestive tract problems that may cause chronic diarrhea include

- celiac disease
- Crohn's disease
- irritable bowel syndrome and other functional gastrointestinal (GI) disorders
- small intestinal bacterial overgrowth
- ulcerative colitis

Abdominal surgery

You may develop chronic diarrhea after abdominal surgery. Abdominal surgery is an operation on the appendix, gallbladder, large intestine, liver, pancreas, small intestine, spleen, or stomach.

Long-term use of medicines

Medicines that must be taken for a long time may cause chronic diarrhea. Some medicines, such as antibiotics, can change the normal gut flora and increase your chances of infection with *Clostridioides difficile*, a bacterium that can cause chronic diarrhea.

How do doctors find the cause of diarrhea?

Doctors do not typically need to find a cause of acute diarrhea. If your diarrhea lasts longer than 4 days or you have symptoms such as fever or bloody stools, your doctor may need to find the cause. Your doctor may use information from your medical and family history, a physical exam, or tests to find the cause of your diarrhea.

Medical and family history

Your doctor will ask for information about your symptoms, such as

- how long you have had diarrhea
- how much stool you have passed
- how often you have diarrhea
- how your stool looks, such as color or consistency
- whether you have other symptoms along with diarrhea

Your doctor will ask about the foods you eat and the beverages you drink. If your doctor suspects you have a food allergy or intolerance, he or she may recommend that you change what you eat to see if your symptoms improve.

Your doctor will also ask about

- current and past medical conditions
- prescription and over-the-counter medicines
- recent contact with other people who are sick
- recent travel to developing countries

Your doctor may ask whether anyone in your family has a history of conditions that cause chronic diarrhea, such as celiac disease, Crohn's disease, irritable bowel syndrome, lactose intolerance, and ulcerative colitis.

Physical exam

During a physical exam, your doctor may

- check your blood pressure and pulse for signs of dehydration
- examine your body for signs of fever or dehydration
- use a stethoscope to listen to sounds in your abdomen
- tap on your abdomen to check for tenderness or pain

Sometimes, doctors perform a digital rectal exam. Your doctor will have you bend over a table or lie on your side while holding your knees close to your chest. After putting on a glove, the doctor will slide a lubricated finger into your anus to check for blood in your stool.

What tests do doctors use to find the cause of diarrhea?

Your doctor may use the following tests to help find the cause of your diarrhea.

Stool test

Stool tests can show the presence of blood, bacteria, or parasites; or signs of diseases and disorders. A health care professional will give you a container for catching and storing the stool. You will receive instructions on where to send or take the container for analysis.

Blood tests

A health care professional may take a blood sample to test for certain diseases or disorders that can cause diarrhea.

Hydrogen breath test

This test is used to diagnose lactose intolerance by measuring the amount of hydrogen in your breath. Normally, little hydrogen is detectable in your breath. With lactose intolerance, undigested lactose produces high levels of hydrogen in your breath. For this test, you will drink a beverage that contains a known amount of lactose. You will then breathe into a balloon-type container that measures your breath hydrogen level. If the hydrogen level is high, your doctor will diagnose lactose intolerance.

Fasting tests

To find out if a food intolerance or allergy is causing your diarrhea, your doctor may ask you to avoid foods with lactose, carbohydrates, wheat, or other ingredients to see whether your diarrhea responds to a change in diet.

Endoscopy

Your doctor may use endoscopy to look inside your body to help find the cause of your diarrhea. Endoscopic procedures include

- colonoscopy
- flexible sigmoidoscopy
- upper gastrointestinal (GI) endoscopy

How can I treat my acute diarrhea?

In most cases, you can treat your acute diarrhea with over-the-counter medicines such as loperamide (Imodium) and bismuth subsalicylate (Pepto-Bismol, Kaopectate). Doctors generally do not recommend using over-the-counter medicines for people who have bloody stools or fever—signs of infection with bacteria or parasites. If your diarrhea lasts more than 2 days, see a doctor right away.

When you have acute diarrhea, you may lose your appetite for a short time. When your appetite returns, you can go back to eating your normal diet. Learn more about eating when you have diarrhea.

How can I treat my child's acute diarrhea?

Over-the-counter medicines to treat acute diarrhea in adults can be dangerous for infants, toddlers, and young children. Talk to a doctor before giving your child an over-the-counter medicine. If your child's diarrhea lasts more than 24 hours, see a doctor right away.

You can give your child his or her usual age-appropriate diet. You can give your infant breast milk or formula as usual.

How do doctors treat persistent and chronic diarrhea?

How doctors treat persistent and chronic diarrhea depends on the cause. Doctors may prescribe antibiotics and medicines that target parasites to treat bacterial or parasitic infections. Doctors may also prescribe medicines to treat some of the conditions that cause chronic diarrhea, such as Crohn's disease, irritable bowel syndrome, or ulcerative colitis. How doctors treat chronic diarrhea in children also depends on the cause.

Doctors may recommend probiotics . Probiotics are live microorganisms, most often bacteria, that are similar to microorganisms you normally have in your digestive tract. Researchers are still studying the use of probiotics to treat diarrhea.

For safety reasons, talk with your doctor before using probiotics or any other complementary or alternative medicines or practices. If your doctor recommends probiotics, talk with him or her about how much probiotics you should take and for how long.

How can I prevent diarrhea?

You can prevent certain types of diarrhea, such as those caused by infections—including rotavirus and traveler's diarrhea—and foodborne illnesses.

Infections

You can reduce your chances of getting or spreading infections that can cause diarrhea by washing your hands thoroughly with soap and warm water for 15 to 30 seconds

- after using the bathroom
- after changing diapers
- before and after handling or preparing food

Rotavirus, which causes viral gastroenteritis, was the

most common cause of diarrhea in infants before rotavirus vaccines became available. The vaccines have reduced the number of cases of rotavirus and hospitalizations due to rotavirus among children in the United States.

Two oral vaccines are approved to protect children from rotavirus infections:

- rotavirus vaccine, live, oral, pentavalent (RotaTeq). Doctors give infants this vaccine in three doses: at 2 months of age, 4 months of age, and 6 months of age.
- rotavirus vaccine, live, oral (Rotarix). Doctors give infants this vaccine in two doses: at 2 months of age and at 4 months of age.

For the rotavirus vaccine to be effective, infants should receive all doses by 8 months of age. Infants 15 weeks of age or older who have never received the rotavirus vaccine should not start the series.

Parents or caregivers of infants should discuss rotavirus vaccination with a doctor.

Travelers' diarrhea

To reduce the chances of getting travelers' diarrhea when traveling to developing countries, avoid

- drinking tap water

- using tap water to make ice, prepare foods or drinks, or brush your teeth
- drinking juice or milk or eating milk products that have not been pasteurized—heated to kill harmful microbes—viruses, bacteria, and parasites
- eating food from street vendors
- eating meat, fish, or shellfish that is raw, undercooked, or not served hot
- eating raw vegetables and most raw fruits

You can drink bottled water, soft drinks, and hot drinks such as coffee or tea made with boiling water.

If you are worried about travelers' diarrhea, talk with your doctor before traveling. Doctors may recommend taking antibiotics before and during a trip to help prevent travelers' diarrhea. Early treatment with antibiotics can shorten a case of travelers' diarrhea.

Foodborne illnesses

You can prevent foodborne illnesses that cause diarrhea by properly storing, cooking, cleaning, and handling foods.

How can I treat or prevent dehydration caused by diarrhea?

To treat or prevent dehydration, you need to replace lost fluids and electrolytes—called rehydration therapy—especially if you have acute diarrhea. Although drinking plenty of water is important in treating and preventing dehydration, you should also drink liquids that contain electrolytes, such as the following:

- broths
- caffeine-free soft drinks
- fruit juices
- sports drinks

If you are an older adult or have a weak immune system, you should also drink oral rehydration solutions, such as Pedialyte, Naturalyte, Infalyte, or CeraLyte. Oral rehydration solutions are liquids that contain glucose and electrolytes. You can make oral rehydration solutions at home (PDF, 90KB) .

How can I treat or prevent my child's dehydration caused by diarrhea?

To treat or prevent dehydration, give your child liquids that contain electrolytes. You can also give your child an oral rehydration solution, such as Pedialyte, Naturalyte, Infalyte, or CeraLyte, as directed. Talk to a doctor about giving these solutions to your infant.

What should I eat if I have diarrhea?

If you have diarrhea, you may lose your appetite for a short time. In most cases, when your appetite returns, you can go back to eating your normal diet. Parents and caretakers should give children with diarrhea their usual age-appropriate diet and give infants breast milk or formula.

Your doctor may recommend changing your diet to treat some causes of chronic diarrhea, such as lactose intolerance or celiac disease.

What should I avoid eating if I have diarrhea?

You should avoid foods that may make your diarrhea worse, such as

- alcoholic beverages
- drinks and foods containing caffeine
- dairy products such as milk, cheese, and ice cream
- fatty and greasy foods
- drinks and foods containing fructose
- fruits such as apples, peaches, and pears
- spicy foods
- diet drinks and sugarless gum and candies containing sweeteners such as sorbitol, mannitol, and xylitol

Research shows that following a restricted diet does

not help treat diarrhea in most cases. Most experts do not recommend fasting or following a restricted diet when you have diarrhea.

Appendix A: Guide to Better Living

Note: Always consult your physician before making any changes to your diet, physical activity or life style.

Is your health condition requires that you make changes to your diet, physical activity, or life style? Are you thinking about being more active? Have you been trying to cut back on less healthy foods? Are you starting to eat better and move more but having a hard time sticking with these changes?

Old habits die hard. Changing your habits is a process that involves several stages. Sometimes it takes a while before changes become new habits. And, you may face roadblocks along the way.

Adopting new, healthier habits may protect you from serious health problems. New habits, like healthy eating and regular physical activity, may also help you manage your weight and have more energy. After a while, if you stick with these changes, they may become part of your daily routine.

The information below outlines four stages you may go through when changing your health habits or behavior. You will also find tips to help you improve your eating, physical activity habits, and overall health. The four stages of changing a health behavior are

- contemplation
- preparation
- action
- maintenance

What stage of change are you in?

Contemplation: "I'm thinking about it."

In this first stage, you are thinking about change and becoming motivated to get started.

You might be in this stage if you

- have been considering change but are not quite ready to start
- believe that your health, energy level, or overall well-being will improve if you develop new habits
- are not sure how you will overcome the roadblocks that may keep you from starting to change

Preparation: "I have made up my mind to take action."

In this next stage, you are making plans and

thinking of specific ideas that will work for you.

You might be in this stage if you

- have decided that you are going to change and are ready to take action
- have set some specific goals that you would like to meet
- are getting ready to put your plan into action

Action: "I have started to make changes."

In this third stage, you are acting on your plan and making the changes you set out to achieve.

You might be in this stage if you

- have been making eating, physical activity, and other behavior changes in the last 6 months or so
- are adjusting to how it feels to eat healthier, be more active, and make other changes such as getting more sleep or reducing screen time
- have been trying to overcome things that sometimes block your success

Maintenance: "I have a new routine."

In this final stage, you have become used to your changes and have kept them up for more than 6 months.

You might be in this stage if

- your changes have become a normal part of your routine
- you have found creative ways to stick with your routine
- you have had slip-ups and setbacks but have been able to get past them and make progress

Did you find your stage of change? Read on for ideas about what you can do next.

Contemplation: Are you thinking of making changes?

Making the leap from thinking about change to taking action can be hard and may take time. Asking yourself about the pros (benefits) and cons (things that get in the way) of changing your habits may be helpful. How would life be better if you made some changes?

Think about how the benefits of healthy eating or regular physical activity might relate to your overall health. For example, suppose your blood glucose, also called blood sugar, is a bit high and you have a parent, brother, or sister who has type 2 diabetes. This means you also may develop type 2 diabetes. You may find that it is easier to be physically active and eat healthy knowing that it may help control blood glucose and protect you from a serious disease.

You may learn more about the benefits of changing your eating and physical activity habits from a health care professional. This knowledge may help you take action.

Look at the lists of pros and cons below. Find the items you believe are true for you. Think about factors that are important to you.

Healthy Eating

Pros	**Cons**
• have more energy	• may spend more money and time on food
• improve my health	• may need to cook more often at home
• lower my risk for health problems	• may need to eat less of foods I love
• maintain a healthy weight	• may need to buy different foods
• feel proud of myself	• may need to convince my family that we all have to eat healthier foods
• set an example for friends and family	

Physical Activity

Pros

- improve my health
- reduce my risk for serious health problems
- feel better about myself
- become stronger
- have fun
- take time to care for myself
- meet new people and spend time with them
- have more energy
- maintain a healthy weight
- become a role model for others

Cons

- takes too much time and energy
- it is too hot or cold outside
- feel self-conscious
- am nervous about my health
- could hurt myself
- am not good at being active
- do not know what to do
- have no one to be active with
- am not young or fit enough
- keeps me from family and friends

Preparation: Have you made up your mind?

If you are in the preparation stage, you are about to take action. To get started, look at your list of pros and cons. How can you make a plan and act on it?

The chart below lists common roadblocks you may face and possible solutions to overcome roadblocks as you begin to change your habits. Think about these things as you make your plan.

Roadblock: I don't have time.

Solution: Make your new healthy habit a priority. Fit in physical activity whenever and wherever you can. Try taking the stairs or getting off the bus a stop early if it is safe to do so. Set aside one grocery shopping day a week, and make healthy meals that you can freeze and eat later when you don't have time to cook.

Roadblock: Healthy habits cost too much.

Solution: You can walk around the mall, a school track, or a local park for free. Eat healthy on a budget by buying in bulk and when items are on sale, and by choosing frozen or canned fruits and vegetables.

Roadblock: I can't make this change alone.

Solution: Recruit others to be active with you, which will help you stay motivated and safe. Consider signing up for a fun fitness class like salsa dancing. Get your family or coworkers on the healthy eating bandwagon. Plan healthy meals together with your family, or start a healthy potluck once a week at work.

Roadblock: I don't like physical activity.

Solution: Forget the old notion that being physically active means lifting weights in a gym. You can be active in many ways, including dancing, walking, or gardening. Make your own list of options that appeal to you. Explore options you never thought about, and stick with what you enjoy.

Roadblock: I don't like healthy foods.

Solution: Try making your old favorite recipes in healthier new ways. For example, you can trim fat from meats and reduce the amount of butter, sugar, and salt you cook with. Use low-fat cheeses or milk rather than whole-milk foods. Add a cup or two of broccoli, carrots, or spinach to casseroles or pasta.

Once you have made up your mind to change your habits, make a plan and set goals for taking action. Here are some ideas for making your plan:

- learn more about healthy eating (https://www.myplate.gov/)
- learn more about being active (see appendix B)
- make lists of
    - healthy foods that you like or may need to eat more of—or more often
    - foods you love that you may need to eat less often
    - things you could do to be more physically active
    - fun activities you like and could do more often, such as dancing

After making your plan, start setting goals for putting your plan into action. Start with small changes. For example, "I'm going to walk for 10 minutes, three times a week." What is the one step you can take right away?

Action: Have you started to make changes?

You are making real changes to your lifestyle, which is fantastic! To stick with your new habits

- review your plan
- look at the goals you set and how well you are meeting them
- overcome roadblocks by planning ahead for setbacks
- reward yourself for your hard work

Track your progress

- Tracking your progress helps you spot your strengths, find areas where you can improve, and stay on course. Record not only what you did, but how you felt while doing it—your feelings can play a role in making your new habits stick.
- Recording your progress may help you stay focused and catch setbacks in meeting your goals. Remember that a setback does not mean you have failed. All of us experience setbacks. The key is to get back on track as soon as you can.
- You can track your progress with online tools such as the NIH Body Weight Planner (https://www.youtube.com/watch?v=v1gluQwi eog). The NIH Body Weight Planner lets you tailor your calorie and physical activity plans to reach your personal goals within a specific time period.

Overcome roadblocks

- Remind yourself why you want to be healthier. Perhaps you want the energy to play with your nieces and nephews or to be able to carry your own grocery bags. Recall your reasons for making changes when slip-ups occur. Decide to take the first step to get back on track.

- Problem-solve to "outsmart" roadblocks. For example, plan to walk indoors, such as at a mall, on days when bad weather keeps you from walking outside.
- Ask a friend or family member for help when you need it, and always try to plan ahead. For example, if you know that you will not have time to be physically active after work, go walking with a coworker at lunch or start your day with an exercise video.

Reward yourself

- After reaching a goal or milestone, allow for a nonfood reward such as new workout gear or a new workout device. Also consider posting a message on social media to share your success with friends and family.
- Choose rewards carefully. Although you should be proud of your progress, keep in mind that a high-calorie treat or a day off from your activity routine are not the best rewards to keep you healthy.
- Pat yourself on the back. When negative thoughts creep in, remind yourself how much good you are doing for your health by moving more and eating healthier.

Maintenance: Have you created a new routine?

Make your future a healthy one. Remember that eating healthy, getting regular physical activity, and other healthy habits are lifelong behaviors, not one-time events. Always keep an eye on your efforts and seek ways to deal with the planned and unplanned changes in life.

Now that healthy eating and regular physical activity are part of your routine, keep things interesting, avoid slip-ups, and find ways to cope with what life throws at you.

Add variety and stay motivated

Mix up your routine with new physical activities and goals, physical activity buddies, foods, recipes, and rewards.

Deal with unexpected setbacks

Plan ahead to avoid setbacks. For example, find other ways to be active in case of bad weather, injury, or other issues that arise. Think of ways to eat healthy when traveling or dining out, like packing healthy snacks while on the road or sharing an entrée with a friend in a restaurant.

If you do have a setback, don't give up. Setbacks happen to everyone. Regroup and focus on meeting your goals again as soon as you can.

Challenge yourself!

Revisit your goals and think of ways to expand them. For example, if you are comfortable walking 5 days a week, consider adding strength training twice a week. If you have limited your saturated fat intake by eating less fried foods, try cutting back on added sugars, too. Small changes can lead to healthy habits worth keeping.

**When The Going Gets Tough,
Put One Foot in Front of The
Other and Just Keep Going.
Don't Give Up!**

Appendix B: How to Stay Active

Note: Always consult your physician before making any changes to your diet, physical activity or life style.

Physical activity may seem hard if you're overweight. You may get short of breath or tired quickly. Finding or affording the right clothes and equipment may be frustrating. Or, perhaps you may not feel comfortable working out in front of others.

The good news is you can overcome these challenges. Not only can you be active at any size, you can have fun and feel good at the same time.

Can anyone be active?

Research strongly shows that physical activity is safe for almost everyone. The health benefits of physical activity far outweigh the risks.

The activities discussed here are safe for most people. If you have problems moving or staying steady on your feet, or if you get out of breath easily, talk with a health care professional before you start. You also should talk with a health care professional if you are unsure of your health, have any concerns that physical activity may be unsafe for you, or have

- a chronic disease such as diabetes, high blood pressure, or heart disease
- a bone or joint problem—for example, in your back, knee, or hip—that could get worse if you change your physical activity level

Why should I be active?

Being active may help you live longer and protect you from developing serious health problems, such as type 2 diabetes, heart disease, stroke, and certain types of cancer. Regular physical activity is linked to many health benefits, such as

- lower blood pressure and blood glucose, or blood sugar
- healthy bones, muscles, and joints
- a strong heart and lungs
- better sleep at night and improved mood

The Physical Activity Guidelines for Americans define regular physical activity as at least 150 minutes a week of moderate-intensity aerobic activity, such as brisk walking. Brisk walking is a pace of 3 miles per hour or faster. A moderate-intensity activity makes you breathe harder but does not overwork or overheat you. You should also do muscle-strengthening activities at least 2 days a week.

You may reach this goal by starting with 5 minutes

of physical activity several times a day, 5 to 6 days a week. You could then gradually work up to 10 minutes per session, 3 times a day. If you do even more activity, you may gain even more health benefits.

When combined with healthy eating, regular physical activity may also help you control your weight. However, research shows that even if you can't lose weight or maintain your weight loss, you still can enjoy important health benefits from regular physical activity.

Physical activity also can be a lot of fun if you do activities you enjoy and are active with other people. Being active with others may give you a chance to meet new people or spend more time with family and friends. You also may inspire and motivate one another to get and stay active.

What do I need to know about becoming active?

Choosing physical activities that match your fitness level and health goals can help you stay motivated and keep you from getting hurt. You may feel some minor discomfort or muscle soreness when you first become active. These feelings should go away as you get used to your activity. However, if you feel sick to your stomach or have pain, you may have done too much. Go easier and then slowly build up your activity level. Some activities, such as walking or swimming, are less likely to cause injuries.

If you have been inactive, start slowly and see how you feel. Gradually increase how long and how often you are active. If you need guidance, check with a health care or certified fitness professional.

Here are some tips for staying safe during physical activity:

- Wear the proper safety gear, such as a bike helmet if you are bicycling.
- Make sure any sports equipment you use works and fits properly.
- Look for safe places to be active. For instance, walk in well-lit areas where other people are around. Be active with a friend or group.
- Stay hydrated to replace the body fluids you lose through sweating and to prevent you from getting overheated.
- If you are active outdoors, protect yourself from the sun with sunscreen and a hat or protective visor and clothing.
- Wear enough clothing to keep warm in cold or windy weather. Layers are best.

If you don't feel right, stop your activity. If you have any of the following warning signs, stop and seek help right away:

- pain, tightness, or pressure in your chest or neck, shoulder, or arm
- extreme shortness of breath
- dizziness or sickness

Check with a health care professional about what to do if you have any of these warning signs. If your activity is causing pain in your joints, feet, ankles, or legs, you also should consult a health care professional to see if you may need to change the type or amount of activity you are doing.

What kinds of activities can I do?

You don't need to be an athlete or have special skills or equipment to make physical activity part of your life. Many types of activities you do every day, such as walking your dog or going up and down steps at home or at work, may help improve your health.

Try different activities you enjoy. If you like an activity, you're more likely to stick with it. Anything that gets you moving around, even for a few minutes at a time, is a healthy start to getting fit.

Walking

Walking is free and easy to do—and you can do it

almost anywhere. Walking will help you

- burn calories
- improve your fitness
- lift your mood
- strengthen your bones and muscles

If you are concerned about safety, try walking in a shopping mall or park where it is well lit and other people are around. Many malls and parks have benches where you can take a quick break. Walking with a friend or family member is safer than walking alone and may provide the social support you need to meet your activity goals.

If you don't have time for a long walk, take several short walks instead. For example, instead of a 30-minute walk, add three 10-minute walks to your day. Shorter spurts of activity are easier to fit into a busy schedule.

Walking tips

- Wear comfortable, well-fitting walking shoes with a lot of support, and socks that absorb sweat.
- Dress for the weather if you are walking outdoors. In cold weather, wear layers of clothing you can remove if you start getting too warm. In hot weather, protect yourself against the sun and heat.

- Warm up by walking more slowly for the first few minutes. Cool down by slowing your pace.

Dancing

Dancing can be a lot of fun while it tones your muscles, strengthens your heart and lungs, and boosts your mood. You can dance at a health club, dance studio, or even at home. Just turn on some lively music and start moving. You also can dance to a video on your TV or computer.

If you have trouble standing on your feet for a long time, try dancing while sitting down. Chair dancing lets you move your arms and legs to music while taking the weight off your feet.

Bicycling

Riding a bicycle spreads your weight among your arms, back, and hips. For outdoor biking, you may want to try a mountain bike. Mountain bikes have wider tires and are sturdier than bikes with thinner tires. You can buy a larger seat to make biking more comfortable.

For indoor biking, you may want to try a recumbent bike. On this type of bike, you sit lower to the ground with your legs reaching forward to the pedals. Your body is in more of a reclining position, which may feel better than sitting straight up. The seat on a recumbent bike is also wider than the seat on a regular bike.

If you decide to buy a bike, check how much weight it can support to make sure it is safe for you.

Workout clothing tips

- Clothes made of fabrics that absorb sweat are best for working out.
- Comfortable, lightweight clothes allow you to move more easily.
- Tights or spandex shorts are the best bottoms to wear to prevent inner-thigh chafing.
- Women should wear a bra that provides extra support during physical activity.

Water workouts

Swimming and water workouts put less stress on your joints than walking, dancing, or biking. If your feet, back, or joints hurt when you stand, water activities may be best for you. If you feel self-conscious about wearing a bathing suit, you can wear shorts and a T-shirt while you swim.

Exercising in water

- Lets you be more flexible. You can move your body in water in ways you may not be able to on land.

- Reduces your risk of hurting yourself. Water provides a natural cushion, which keeps you from pounding or jarring your joints.
- Helps prevent sore muscles.
- Keeps you cool, even when you are working hard.

You don't need to know how to swim to work out in water. You can do shallow- or deep-water exercises at either end of the pool without swimming. For instance, you can do laps while holding onto a kickboard and kicking your feet. You also can walk or jog across the width of the pool while moving your arms.

For shallow-water workouts, the water level should be between your waist and chest. During deep-water workouts, most of your body is underwater. For safety and comfort, wear a foam belt or life jacket.

Tips for protecting your hair

If you're worried that pool water will damage or mess up your hair, try these tips:

- Use a swim cap to help protect your hair from pool chemicals and getting wet.
- Wear a natural hairstyle, short braids, locs, or twists, which may be easier to style after a water workout.

- Buy a shampoo to remove chlorine buildup, available at most drug stores, if your hair feels dry or damaged after a pool workout.

Strength training

Strength training involves using free weights, weightlifting machines, resistance bands, or your own body weight to make your muscles stronger. Lower-body strength training will improve your balance and prevent falls.

Strength training may help you

- build and maintain strong muscles as you get older
- continue to perform activities of daily living, such as carrying groceries or moving furniture
- keep your bones strong, which may help prevent osteoporosis and fractures

If you arc just starting out, using a weightlifting machine may be safer than dumbbells. As you get fit, you may want to add free-weight exercises with dumbbells.

You do not need a weight bench or large dumbbells to do strength training at home. You can use a pair of hand weights to do bicep curls. You can also use your own body weight: for example, get up and down from a chair.

Proper form is very important when lifting weights. You may hurt yourself if you don't lift weights properly. You may want to schedule a session with a certified fitness professional to learn which exercises to do and how to do them safely. Check with your health insurer about whether your health plan covers these services.

If you decide to buy a home gym, check how much weight it can support to make sure it is safe for you.

Strength-training tips

- Aim for at least 2 days per week of strengthen-training activities.
- Try to perform each exercise 8 to 12 times. If that's too hard, the weight you are lifting is too heavy. If it's too easy, your weight is too light.
- Try to exercise all the major muscle groups. These groups include the muscles of the legs, hips, chest, back, abdomen, shoulders, and arms.
- Don't work the same muscles 2 days in a row. Your muscles need time to recover.

Mind and body exercise

Your local hospital or fitness, recreation, or community center may offer classes such as yoga, tai chi, or Pilates. You also may find some of these workouts online and can download them to a computer, smart phone, or other device. These types of activities may help you

- become stronger and more flexible
- feel more relaxed
- improve balance and posture

Your local hospital or fitness, recreation, or community center may offer classes such as yoga, tai chi, or Pilates.

These classes also can be a lot of fun and add variety to your workout routine. If some movements are hard to do or you have injuries you are concerned about, talk with the instructor about how to adapt the exercises and poses to meet your needs—or start with a beginner's class.

Daily life activities

Daily life activities, such as cleaning out the attic or washing the car, are great ways to get moving. Small changes can add more physical activity to your day and improve your health. Try these:

- Take 2- to 3-minute walking breaks at work several times a day, if possible.
- Stand, walk, or stretch in place during TV commercials.
- Take the stairs instead of the elevator or escalator whenever you can.

- Park farther from where you are going and walk the rest of the way.

Even a shopping trip can be exercise because it provides a chance to walk and carry your bags. Chores such as mowing the lawn, raking leaves, and gardening also count.

Where can I be active?

You can find many fun places to be active. Having more than one place may keep you from getting bored. Here are some options:

- Join or take a class at a local fitness, recreation, or community center.
- Enjoy the outdoors by taking a hike or going for a walk in a safe local park, neighborhood, or mall.
- Work out in the comfort of your own home with a workout video or by finding a fitness channel on your TV, tablet, or other mobile device.

Tips for choosing a fitness center

- Make sure the center has exercise equipment for people who weigh more and staff to show you how to use it.
- Ask if the center has any special classes for people just starting out, older adults, or people with mobility or health issues.

- See if you can try out the center or take a class before you join.
- Try to find a center close to work or home. The quicker and easier the center is to get to, the better your chances of using it often.
- Make sure you understand the rules for joining and ending your membership, what your membership fee covers, any related costs, and the days and hours of operation.

How can I get past my roadblocks?

You most likely will face roadblocks that keep you from meeting your physical activity goals. Think about what keeps you from being active, then try to come up with creative ways to address those roadblocks. Here are a few examples to help you get started:

Barrier: I don't have enough time.

Solution: Instead of doing one long workout session, build in three 10-minute bursts of activity during your day, such as a brisk walk. Even standing up instead of sitting at your desk has benefits.

Barrier: I just don't like exercise.

Solution: Good news! You don't have to run a marathon or go to the gym all the time to benefit from being active. To make physical activity more fun, try something you enjoy doing, such as dancing to the radio or taking a yoga class with friends. Many people find they start to like exercise better the more they do it.

Barrier: I'm worried about my health or getting hurt.

Solution: If you have a hard time being active because of your health, talk with a health care professional first. A certified fitness professional can also guide you on how to be active safely.

Barrier: I feel self-conscious working out in front of others.

Solution: Start being active at home until you feel more confident. Be active with friends who will support and encourage you.

How can I stick with my physical activity plan?

Sticking with a plan to be physically active can be a challenge. Online tools such as the NIH Body Weight Planner (https://www.youtube.com/watch?v=v1gluQwieog) can help. The NIH Body Weight Planner lets you tailor your calorie and physical activity plans to reach your personal goals within a specific time period.

You also can download fitness apps that let you enter information to track your progress using a computer or smart phone or other mobile device.

Devices you can wear, such as pedometers and fitness trackers, may help you count steps, calories, and minutes of physical activity. Trackers can help you set goals and monitor progress. You wear most of these devices on your wrist like a watch, or clipped to your clothing.

Keeping an activity journal is another good way to help you stay motivated and on track to reach your fitness goals.

Set goals. As you track your activity, try to set specific short- and long-term goals. For example, instead of "I will be more active," set a goal such as "I will take a walk after lunch at least 2 days a week." Getting started with a doable goal is a good way to form a new habit. A short-term goal may be to walk 5 to 10 minutes, 5 days a week. A long-term goal may be to do at least 150 minutes of moderate-intensity physical activity a week.

Get support. Ask a family member or friend to be active with you. Your workout buddy can help make your activities more fun and can cheer you on and help you meet your goals.

Track progress. You may not feel as though you

are making progress, but when you look back at where you started, you may be pleasantly surprised. Making regular activity part of your life is a big step. Start slowly and praise yourself for every goal you set and achieve.

Review your goals. Did you meet your goals? If not, why? Are they doable? Did you hit a roadblock trying to meet your goal? What will you do differently next week? Brainstorm some options to overcome future roadblocks. Ask a friend or family member to help support your goals.

Pick nonfood rewards. Whether your goal is to be active 15 minutes a day, to walk farther than you did last week, or simply to stay positive, recognizing your efforts is an important part of staying on track. Decide how you will reward yourself. Some ideas for rewards include getting new music to charge you up or buying new workout gear.

Be patient with yourself. Don't get discouraged if you have setbacks from time to time. If you can't achieve your goal the first time or can only stick to your goals for part of the week, remind yourself that this is all part of establishing new habits.

Look ahead. Try to focus on what you will do differently moving forward, rather than on what went wrong. Pat yourself on the back for trying.

Most importantly, don't give up. Any movement, even for a short time, is a good thing. Each activity you add to your life is another step toward a healthier you.